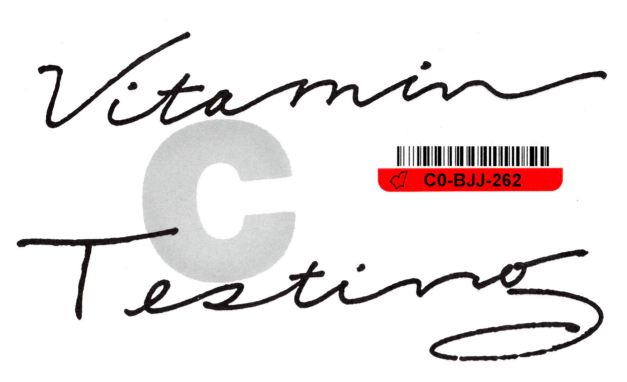

Vitamin C Testing

Grades 4–8

Skills

Chemistry Laboratory Techniques,
Experimenting, Analyzing Data, Graphing,
Drawing Conclusions

Concepts

Vitamin C Content, Nutrition,
Titration, Indicator, End Point,
Conditions Causing Vitamin Loss

Themes

Change, Stability, Equilibrium,
Systems, Interactions

Time

Four 45-minute sessions
plus follow-up sessions

Jacqueline Barber

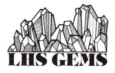

LHS GEMS

Great Explorations in Math and Science (GEMS)
Lawrence Hall of Science
University of California at Berkeley

Illustrations
Carol Bevilacqua

Photographs
Jacqueline Barber
Richard Hoyt

Lawrence Hall of Science, University of California,
Berkeley, CA 94720
© 1988 by The Regents of the University of California.
All rights reserved. Printed in the United States of
America. Reprinted with revisions, 1990.

International Standard Book Number: 0-912511-70-2.

Publication was made possible by grants from the A. W.
Mellon Foundation and the Carnegie Corporation of
New York. GEMS also gratefully acknowledges the
contribution of word processing equipment from Apple
Computer, Inc.

COMMENTS WELCOME

Great Explorations in Math and Science (GEMS) is
an ongoing curriculum development project. GEMS
Guides are revised periodically, to incorporate
teacher comments and new approaches. We
welcome your criticisms, suggestions, helpful hints,
and any anecdotes about your experience
presenting GEMS activities. Your suggestions will
be reviewed each time a GEMS Guide is revised.
Please send your comments to: GEMS Revisions,
c/o Lawrence Hall of Science, University of
California, Berkeley, CA 94720.

Great Explorations in Math and Science (GEMS) Project

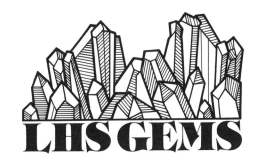

The Lawrence Hall of Science (LHS) is a public science center on the University of California at Berkeley campus. LHS offers a full program of activities for the public, including films, lectures, special events, exhibits, classes and workshops. LHS is also a center for teacher training and curriculum research and development.

Over the years, LHS staff have developed a number of activities, assembly programs, classes and exhibits. These programs have proved to be successful at the Hall and should be useful to other science centers, museums, schools, and community groups. Grants from the A. W. Mellon Foundation and the Carnegie Corporation of New York have made possible the publication of these activities under the "Great Explorations in Math and Science" (GEMS) title.

Staff

Glenn T. Seaborg, **Principal Investigator**
Robert C. Knott, **Administrator**
Jacqueline Barber, **Director**

Cynthia Ashley, Administrative Coordinator
Lisa Haderlie Baker, Art Director
Carol Bevilacqua and Lisa Klofkorn, Designers
Lincoln Bergman and Kay Fairwell, Editors
Betsy Ross, Administrative Assistant

Contributing Authors

Leigh Agler
Jeremy Ahouse
Jacqueline Barber
Katharine Barrett
Lincoln Bergman
Marion E. Buegler
David Buller
Linda De Lucchi
Jean Echols
Alan Gould
Cheryll Hawthorne
Jefferey Kaufmann
Robert C. Knott
Larry Malone
Cary I. Sneider
Elizabeth Stage

Reviewers

We would like to thank the following educators who reviewed, tested, or coordinated the reviewing of this series of GEMS materials in manuscript form. Their critical comments and recommendations contributed significantly to these GEMS publications. Their participation does not necessarily imply endorsement of the GEMS program.

ARIZONA

David P. Anderson
Royal Palm Junior High School, Phoenix

Joanne Anger
John Jacobs Elementary School, Phoenix

Cheri Balkenbush
Shaw Butte Elementary School, Phoenix

Flo-Ann Barwick Campbell
Mountain Sky Junior High School, Phoenix

Sandra Caldwell
Lakeview Elementary School, Phoenix

Richard Clark*
Washington School District, Phoenix

Kathy Culbertson
Moon Mountain Elementary School, Phoenix

Don Diller
Sunnyslope Elementary School, Phoenix

Barbara G. Elliot
Tumbleweed Elementary School, Phoenix

Joseph M. Farrier
Desert Foothills Junior High School, Phoenix

Mary Anne French
Moon Mountain Elementary School, Phoenix

Leo H. Hamlet
Desert View Elementary School, Phoenix

Elaine Hardt
Sunnyslope Elementary School, Phoenix

Walter Carroll Hart
Desert View Elementary School, Phoenix

Tim Huff
Sunnyslope Elementary School, Phoenix

Stephen H. Kleinz
Desert Foothills Junior High School, Phoenix

Alison Lamborghini
Orangewood Elementary School, Phoenix

Karen Lee
Moon Mountain Elementary School, Phoenix

George Lewis
Sweetwater Elementary School, Phoenix

Tom Lutz
Palo Verde Junior High School, Phoenix

Midori Mits
Sunset Elementary School, Phoenix

Brenda Pierce
Cholla Junior High School, Phoenix

Sue Poe
Palo Verde Junior High School, Phoenix

Robert C. Rose
Sweetwater Elementary School, Phoenix

Liz Sandberg
Desert Foothills Junior High School, Phoenix

Jacque Sniffen
Chaparral Elementary School, Phoenix

Rebecca Staley
John Jacobs Elementary School, Phoenix

Sandra Stanley
Manzanita Elementary School, Phoenix

Chris Starr
Sunset Elementary School, Phoenix

Karen R. Stock
Tumbleweed Elementary School, Phoenix

Charri L. Strong
Mountain Sky Junior High School, Phoenix

Shirley Vojtko
Cholla Junior High School, Phoenix

K. Dollar Wroughton
John Jacobs Elementary School, Phoenix

CALIFORNIA

Carolyn R. Adams
Washington Primary School, Berkeley

Judith Adler*
Walnut Heights Elementary School, Walnut Creek

Gretchen P. Anderson
Buena Vista Elementary School, Walnut Creek

Beverly Braxton
Columbus Intermediate School, Berkeley

Dorothy Brown
Cave Elementary School, Vallejo

Christa Buckingham
Seven Hills Intermediate School, Walnut Creek

Elizabeth Burch
Sleepy Hollow Elementary School, Orinda

Katharine V. Chapple
Walnut Heights Elementary School, Walnut Creek

Linda Clar
Walnut Heights Elementary School, Walnut Creek

Gail E. Clarke
The Dorris-Eaton School, Walnut Creek

Sara J. Danielson
Albany Middle School, Albany

Robin Davis
Albany Middle School, Albany

Margaret Dreyfus
Walnut Heights Elementary School, Walnut Creek

Jose Franco
Columbus Intermediate School, Berkeley

Elaine Gallaher
Sleepy Hollow Elementary School, Orinda

Ann Gilbert
Columbus Intermediate School, Berkeley

Gretchen Gillfillan
Sleepy Hollow Elementary School, Orinda

Brenda S.K. Goo
Cave Elementary School, Vallejo

Beverly Kroske Grunder
Indian Valley Elementary School, Walnut Creek

Kenneth M. Guthrie
Walnut Creek Intermediate School, Walnut Creek

Joan Hedges
Walnut Heights Elementary School, Walnut Creek

Corrine Howard
Washington Elementary School, Berkeley

Janet Kay Howard
Sleepy Hollow Elementary School, Orinda

Gail Isserman
Murwood Elementary School, Walnut Creek

Carol Jensen
Columbus Intermediate School, Berkeley

Dave Johnson
Cave Elementary School, Vallejo

Kathy Jones
Cave Elementary School, Vallejo

Dayle Kerstad*
Cave Elementary School, Vallejo

Diane Knickerbocker
Indian Valley Elementary School, Walnut Creek

Joan P. Kunz
Walnut Heights Elementary School, Walnut Creek

Randy Lam
Los Cerros Intermediate School, Danville

Philip R. Loggins
Sleepy Hollow Elementary School, Orinda

Jack McFarland
Albany Middle School, Albany

Betty Maddox
Walnut Heights Elementary School, Walnut Creek

Chiyomi Masuda
Columbus Intermediate School, Berkeley

Katy Miles
Albany Middle School, Albany

Lin Morehouse*
Sleepy Hollow Elementary Schoool, Orinda

Marv Moss
Sleepy Hollow Elementary School, Orinda

Tina L. Neivelt
Cave Elementary School, Vallejo

Neil Nelson
Cave Elementary School, Vallejo

Joyce Noakes
Valle Verde Elementary School, Walnut Creek

Jill Norris
Sleepy Hollow Elementary School, Orinda

Janet Obata
Albany Middle School, Albany

Patrick Pase
Los Cerros Intermediate School, Danville

Geraldine Piglowski
Cave Elementary School, Vallejo

Susan Power
Albany Middle School, Albany

Louise Rasmussen
Albany Middle School, Albany

Jan Rayder
Columbus Intermediate School, Berkeley

Masha Rosenthal
Sleepy Hollow Elementary School, Orinda

Carol Rutherford
Cave Elementary School, Vallejo

Jim Salak
Cave Elementary School, Vallejo

Constance M. Schulte
Seven Hills Intermediate School, Walnut Creek

Robert Shogren*
Albany Middle School, Albany

Kay L. Sorg*
Albany Middle School, Albany

Marc Tatar
University of California Gifted Program, Berkeley

Mary E. Welte
Sleepy Hollow Elementary School, Orinda

Carol Whitmore-Waldron
Cave Elementary School, Vallejo

Vernola J. Williams
Albany Middle School, Albany

Carolyn Willard*
Columbus Intermediate School, Berkeley

Mary Yonekawa
The Dorris-Eaton School, Walnut Creek

KENTUCKY

Joyce M. Anderson
Carrithers Middle School, Louisville

Susan H. Baker
Museum of History and Science, Louisville

Carol Earle Black
Highland Middle School, Louisville

April B. Bond
Rangeland Elementary School, Louisville

Sue M. Brown
Newburg Middle School, Louisville

Donna Ross Butler
Carrithers Middle School, Louisville

Stacey Cade
Sacred Heart Model School, Louisville

Sister Catherine, O.S.U.
Sacred Heart Model School, Louisville

Judith Kelley Dolt
Gavin H. Cochran Elementary School,
Louisville

Elizabeth Dudley
Carrithers Middle School, Louisville

Jeanne Flowers
Sacred Heart Model School, Louisville

Karen Fowler
Carrithers Middle School, Louisville

Laura Hansen
Sacred Heart Model School, Louisville

Sandy Hill-Binkley
Museum of History and Science, Louisville

Deborah M. Hornback
Museum of History and Science, Louisville

Patricia A. Hulak
Newburg Middle School, Louisville

Rose Isetti
Museum of History and Science, Louisville

Mary Ann M. Kent
Sacred Heart Model School, Louisville

James D. Kramer
Gavin H. Cochran Elementary School,
Louisville

Sheneda Little
Gavin H. Cochran Elementary School,
Louisville

Brenda W. Logan
Newburg Middle School, Louisville

Amy S. Lowen*
Museum of History and Science, Louisville

Mary Louise Marshall
Breckinridge Elementary School, Louisville

Theresa H. Mattei*
Museum of History and Science, Louisville

Judy Reibel
Highland Middle School, Louisville

Pamela R. Record
Highland Middle School, Louisville

Margie Reed
Carrithers Middle School, Louisville

Donna Rice
Carrithers Middle School, Louisville

Ken Rosenbaum
Jefferson County Public Schools, Louisville

Edna Schoenbaechler
Museum of History and Science, Louisville

Karen Schoenbaechler
Museum of History and Science, Louisville

Deborah G. Semenick
Breckinridge Elementary School, Louisville

Dr. William McLean Sudduth*
Museum of History and Science, Louisville

Rhonda H. Swart
Carrithers Middle School, Louisville

Arlene S. Tabor
Gavin H. Cochran Elementary School,
Louisville

Carla M. Taylor
Museum of History and Science, Louisville

Carol A. Trussell
Rangeland Elementary School, Louisville

Janet W. Varon
Newburg Middle School, Louisville

MICHIGAN

Glen Blinn
Harper Creek High School, Battle Creek

Douglas M. Bollone
Kelloggsville Junior High School, Wyoming

Sharon Christensen*
Delton-Kellogg Middle School, Delton

Ruther M. Conner
Parchment Middle School, Kalamazoo

Stirling Fenner
Gull Lake Middle School, Hickory Corners

Dr. Alonzo Hannaford*
Western Michigan University, Kalamazoo

Barbara Hannaford
The Gagie School, Kalamazoo

Duane Hornbeck
St. Joseph Elementary School, Kalamazoo

Mary M. Howard
The Gagie School, Kalamazoo

Diane Hartman Larsen
Plainwell Middle School, Plainwell

Miriam Hughes
Parchment Middle School, Kalamazoo

Dr. Phillip T. Larsen*
Western Michigan University, Kalamazoo

David M. McDill
Harper Creek High School, Battle Creek

Sue J. Molter
Dowagiac Union High School, Dowagiac

Julie Northrop
South Junior High School, Kalamazoo

Judith O'Brien
Dowagiac Union High School, Dowagiac

Rebecca Penney
Harper Creek High School, Battle Creek

Susan C. Popp
Riverside Elementary School, Constantine

Brenda Potts
Riverside Elementary School, Constantine

Karen Prater
St. Joseph Elementary School, Kalamazoo

Joel Schuitema
Woodland Elementary School, Portage

Pete Vunovich
Harper Creek Junior High School, Battle
Creek

Beverly E. Wrubel
Woodland Elementary School, Portage

NEW YORK

Frances P. Bargamian
Trinity Elementary School, New Rochelle

Barbara Carter
Jefferson Elementary School, New Rochelle

Ann C. Faude
Heathcote Elementary School, Scarsdale

Steven T. Frantz
Heathcote Elementary School, Scarsdale

Alice A. Gaskin
Edgewood Elementary School, Scarsdale

Harriet Glick
Ward Elementary School, New Rochelle

Richard Golden*
Barnard School, New Rochelle

Seymour Golden
Albert Leonard Junior High School, New
Rochelle

Don Grant
Isaac E. Young Junior High School, New
Rochelle

Marybeth Greco
Heathcote Elementary School, Scarsdale

Peter C. Haupt
Fox Meadow Elementary School, Scarsdale

Tema Kaufman
Edgewood Elementary School, Scarsdale

Donna MacCrae
Webster Magnet Elementary School, New
Rochelle

Dorothy T. McElroy
Edgewood Elementary School, Scarsdale

Mary Jane Motl
Greenacres Elementary School, Scarsdale

Tom Mullen
Jefferson Elementary School, New Rochelle

Robert Nebens
Ward Elementary School, New Rochelle

Eileen L. Paolicelli
Ward Elementary School, New Rochelle

Donna Pentaleri
Heathcote Elementary School, Scarsdale

Dr. John V. Pozzi*
City School District of New Rochelle, New
Rochelle

John J. Russo
Ward Elementary School, New Rochelle

Bruce H. Seiden
Webster Magnet Elementary School, New
Rochelle

David B. Selleck
Albert Leonard Junior High School, New
Rochelle

Lovelle Stancarone
Trinity Elementary School, New Rochelle

Tina Sudak
Ward Elementary School, New Rochelle

Julia Taibi
Davis Elementary School, New Rochelle

Kathy Vajda
Webster Magnet Elementary School, New
Rochelle

Charles B. Yochim
Davis Elementary School, New Rochelle

Bruce D. Zeller
Isaac E. Young Junior High School, New
Rochelle

DENMARK

Dr. Erik W. Thulstrup
Royal Danish School of Educational Studies,
Copenhagen

*Trial test coordinators

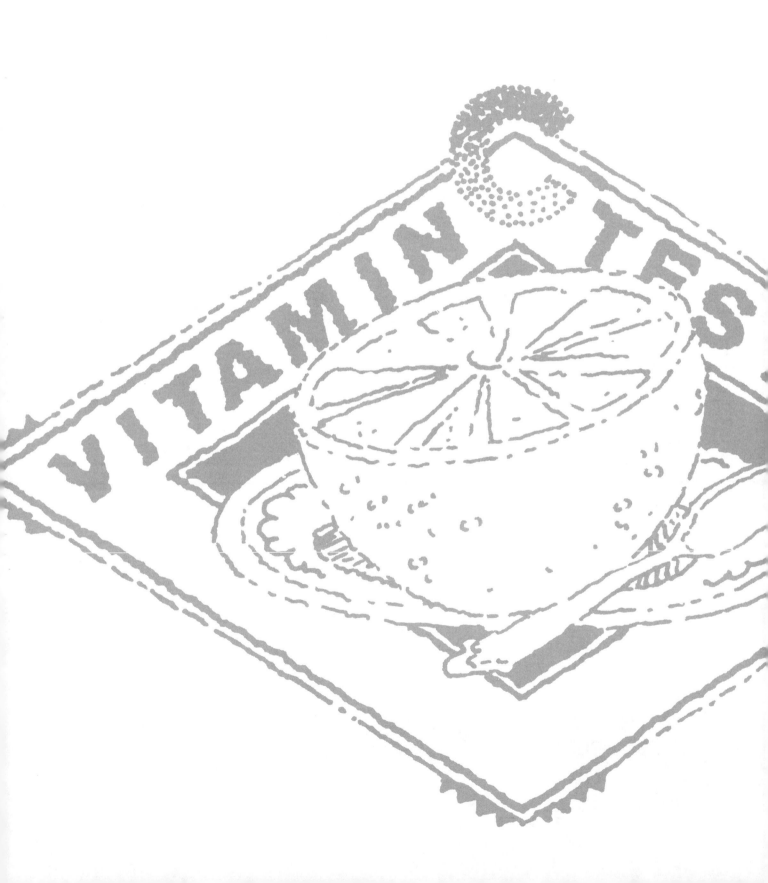

Contents

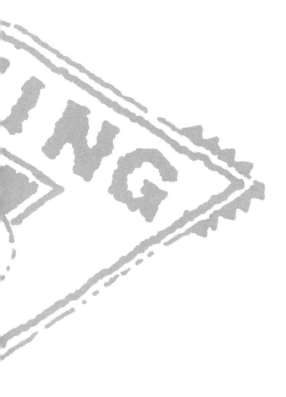

Acknowledgments

Testing for vitamin C content by titration is a standard laboratory technique that was first introduced as an activity for students at the Lawrence Hall of Science by Bonnie King. Over a period of several years, Jacqueline Barber, the author of *Vitamin C Testing*, presented the activities to many classes of students, and developed many of the improvements and extensions that appear in this version. David Buller and other instructors contributed further refinements. Cary Sneider produced the final draft of this GEMS Teacher's Guide.

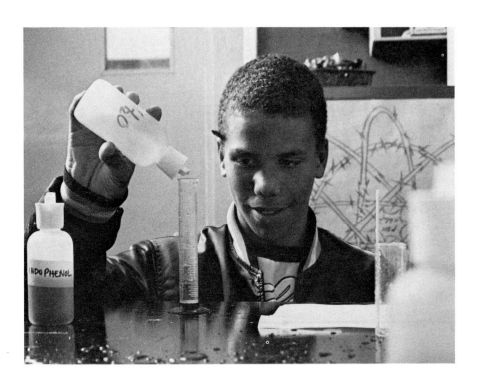

Introduction

"Drink your orange juice every morning—it has lots of vitamin C!" "Drink Brand A apple juice—it's fortified with vitamins!" "Don't boil vegetables—they'll lose their nutritional value!" We hear statements like these from friends and relatives, from the media, and from companies that claim their products are more nutritious than those of the competition. Yet very few people have the opportunity to test these claims for themselves. Vitamin C Testing offers a fun, experimental introduction to chemistry and nutrition by providing your students with the materials and techniques they need to test the vitamin C content in common juices.

In Session 1, the students learn to use a chemical technique called *titration.* The titration involves adding a test beverage, drop-by-drop, to an indicator solution that undergoes a series of color changes as vitamin C is added to it: blue to violet to pink to colorless. As the class begins testing, you'll hear cries of: "Fresh orange juice took five drops!" "Apple juice took 39 drops!" and "This vitamin C solution took only one drop!"

In Session 2, students pool their data, calculate averages, and make a bar graph to represent the class results. They draw conclusions about the relative amounts of vitamin C in juices made from different kinds of fruits, and explore how different processes, such as freezing or canning, can affect vitamin C content.

In Session 3, your students measure the amount of vitamin C in fruit drinks they bring in from home. This allows them to make an important connection between the laboratory tests they perform in school and the nutritional value of liquids they drink every day.

How important is it to put the lid on the juice jar and store it in the refrigerator? In Session 4, your students investigate this question, using the titration technique to conduct experiments on how the treatment of foods affects nutritional value.

Summary Outlines are provided to assist you in guiding your students through these activities in an organized manner. Student data sheets appear immediately following the session in which they are needed. Removable copies of the data sheets are included in the back of the booklet.

Before including *Vitamin C Testing* in this year's science curriculum, you should be aware that:

● All of the materials you will need are available in local stores except for the indicator chemical, indophenol, and plastic vials which must be ordered from a scientific supply company. (See page 43 for a list of suppliers.) Chemicals sometimes take several weeks to ship, so plan ahead!

● *Vitamin C Testing* requires some time to prepare the first time you teach it. **Please see "An Important Note about Preparation" on page 7 for time-saving ideas.**

As with other hands-on science activities, the effort required to plan and present *Vitamin C Testing* will be amply rewarded by the increase in student enthusiasm for and understanding of science. In this unit, chemistry becomes a practical tool your students can use to determine, for themselves, the accuracy of advertising claims, as they gain basic information on nutrition.

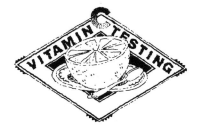

Time Frame

Session 1: Conducting the Tests
      Teacher Preparation: 60 minutes
      Classroom Activity: 45 minutes

Session 2: Analyzing the Results
      Teacher Preparation: 15 minutes
      Classroom Activity: 45 minutes

Session 3: Testing More Beverages
      Teacher Preparation: 20 minutes
      Classroom Activity: 45 minutes

Session 4: Experimenting with Vitamin C Content
      Teacher Preparation: 40 minutes
      Classroom Activity: 30–45 minutes

The preparation times estimated above will vary, depending on the number of juices you plan to include in the tests and whether or not students help you prepare. (Time-saving ideas are listed on page 7.)

The time needed for classroom activities will also vary, depending on the age level of your students and the number of juices they are testing. You may need to continue a session during the next available science period if your students have not finished their laboratory work or discussion.

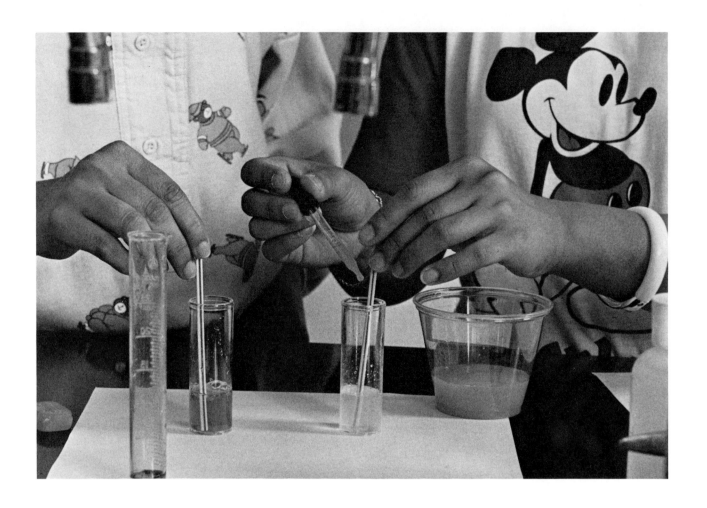

Session 1: Conducting the Tests

Overview

In this session, your students use a laboratory technique called *titration* to test various fruit drinks for relative vitamin C content. Titration involves adding one liquid to another, drop by drop, until a specified outcome, such as a color change, is achieved. The titration in this unit involves an indicator solution named indophenol that undergoes a series of color changes as vitamin C is added to it.

The students add drops of the beverage they are testing to a vial of indophenol solution, and an equal number of drops of the beverage to a control vial containing water. Students record the number of drops required to change the color of the indophenol solution until it becomes the same color as the contents of the control vial. The point at which the contents of the two vials become the same color is called the *end point* of the titration.

The primary objectives of this session are for the students to learn the laboratory procedure for testing relative vitamin C content, and to collect data that will be analyzed in Session 2.

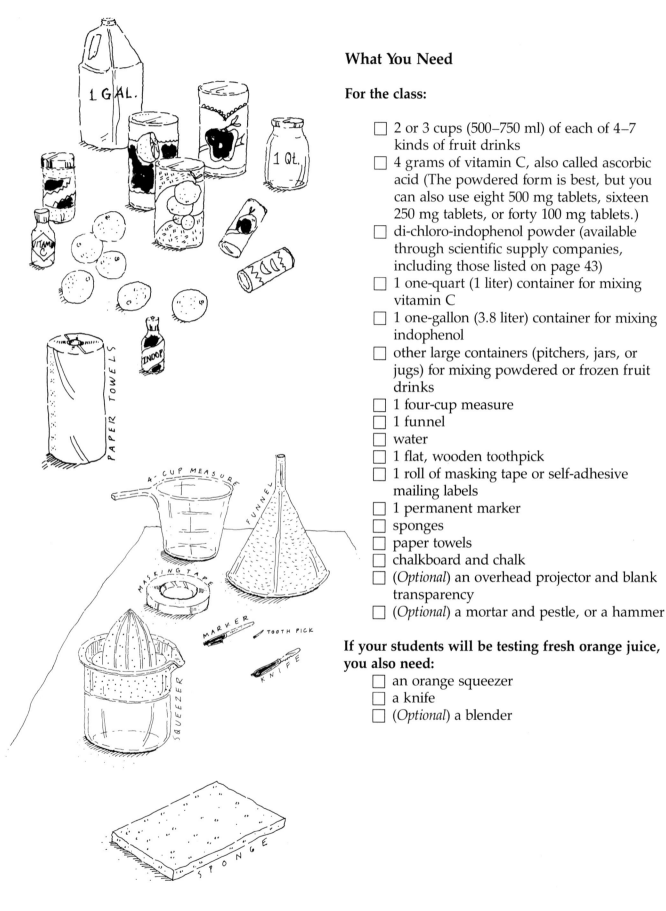

What You Need

For the class:

- ☐ 2 or 3 cups (500–750 ml) of each of 4–7 kinds of fruit drinks
- ☐ 4 grams of vitamin C, also called ascorbic acid (The powdered form is best, but you can also use eight 500 mg tablets, sixteen 250 mg tablets, or forty 100 mg tablets.)
- ☐ di-chloro-indophenol powder (available through scientific supply companies, including those listed on page 43)
- ☐ 1 one-quart (1 liter) container for mixing vitamin C
- ☐ 1 one-gallon (3.8 liter) container for mixing indophenol
- ☐ other large containers (pitchers, jars, or jugs) for mixing powdered or frozen fruit drinks
- ☐ 1 four-cup measure
- ☐ 1 funnel
- ☐ water
- ☐ 1 flat, wooden toothpick
- ☐ 1 roll of masking tape or self-adhesive mailing labels
- ☐ 1 permanent marker
- ☐ sponges
- ☐ paper towels
- ☐ chalkboard and chalk
- ☐ (*Optional*) an overhead projector and blank transparency
- ☐ (*Optional*) a mortar and pestle, or a hammer

If your students will be testing fresh orange juice, you also need:

- ☐ an orange squeezer
- ☐ a knife
- ☐ (*Optional*) a blender

For each group of 4–6 students:

- [ ] 1 cafeteria tray
- [ ] 1 clear plastic wide-mouthed cup for each fruit drink
- [ ] 1 clear plastic cup for the vitamin C solution
- [ ] 1 medicine dropper for each fruit drink and vitamin C
- [ ] 1 large or several small waste containers (e.g., 1 large dishpan or several 12-oz. cottage cheese containers)

For each pair of students:

- [ ] 2 graduated cylinders (for measuring 10 ml quantities)
- [ ] 2 colorless plastic vials (discarded pill containers from hospitals or vials purchased from suppliers listed on page 43)
- [ ] 2 5–10 oz. (250–500 ml) plastic squeeze bottles (Empty hand lotion, shampoo, or dishwashing liquid bottles may be used if they have been thoroughly cleaned.)
- [ ] 2 plastic stir sticks (such as coffee stirrers)
- [ ] 2 8½" x 11" sheets of white paper
- [ ] 2 data sheets (master included on page 17)
- [ ] 2 pencils
- [ ] (*Optional*) 2 pairs of safety goggles

An Important Note about Preparation

The amount of preparation required for this activity is considerable the first time you teach it. Any or all of the following recommendations can help save time:

- Share the tasks with another teacher at your school.

- Have several of your students label containers, fill squeeze bottles, squeeze oranges, pour the fruit drinks into their labeled cups, and arrange the containers on trays. (For preparation details, see the "Getting Ready" sections for each session.)

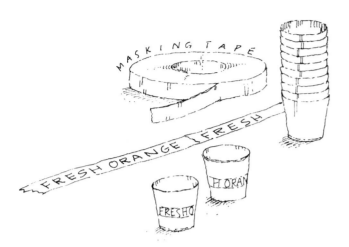

- Labels for containers can be made quickly by one of these methods: (1) Use the master label sheet at the end of this guide to duplicate labels for "Water," "Indophenol Solution," and "Vitamin C Solution" onto a blank sheet of self-adhesive mailing labels. Make your own master and use this same method to make labels for each of the beverages your students will test. (2) Stick several feet of masking tape to a flat, smooth surface and write the name of the solution 4 to 6 times along the strip. Then remove the tape labels piece by piece as you stick them onto the containers.

- If you feel comfortable with a high level of student traffic during testing, you can set up a station for each fruit drink, thus eliminating the need to label cups. At each station, place several cups of the drink and something that will identify it (its can, jar, or paper packaging). Set testing equipment at each station so pairs of students can circulate from station to station with their data sheets. The following instructions assume you will not use stations, but will have lab teams work with their own sets of equipment.

- Rinse the labeled containers after the activity and save them for the next time you present *Vitamin C Testing*.

Getting Ready

Before the Day of the Activity:

1. Purchase Fruit Beverages

Choose a number of orange drinks produced in a variety of ways, such as orange juice that is fresh, frozen, or canned, or orange drinks that are powdered, canned, or vacuum-sealed in foil containers.

Also choose several non-orange juices—such as apple, grapefruit, pineapple, lemonade, or white grape juice—that all have been processed in the same way (canned, frozen, or vacuum-sealed in jars). **Avoid red and purple juices, as their color will obscure the color indication for vitamin C.** If possible, avoid beverages with added vitamin C, which might be described on the list of ingredients as "ascorbic acid."

Testing a variety of orange juices will allow students to draw conclusions about the effect of different processing methods on vitamin C content. Testing juices from different fruits, prepared in the same way, will allow comparison of the vitamin C content in different fruit drinks. However, keep in mind that more juices also mean more time spent in preparation and during the class activity. In Session 3, students will be asked to bring in fruit drinks from home to test.

2. Label Containers.

   a. Label one cup with the name of each beverage and label one cup "Vitamin C Solution" for each group of 4–6 students. See page 8 for labeling shortcuts.

   b. For each pair of students, label one squeeze bottle "Indophenol Solution."

   c. For each pair of students, label one squeeze bottle "Water."

      See the master label sheet at the end of this guide.

3. Prepare Test Juices.

   a. Dissolve 4 grams of vitamin C (ascorbic acid) in about 3 cups (750 ml) of water. Ascorbic acid powder dissolves faster than tablets. Use a mortar and pestle, or a hammer, to crush the tablets if you want them to dissolve immediately. The tablets will dissolve by themselves if left in water for several hours.

b. Prepare powdered and frozen fruit drinks according to the instructions on their packages. Save all packaging in case you decide to follow this series of activities with a lesson on reading labels and analyzing advertising claims. (See "Going Further," page 38.)

4. Prepare the indophenol solution.

PLEASE NOTE: The indophenol solution used in class activities is so dilute that it is safe for students to use. However, the concentrated powder can be harmful, and **you should be careful not to get the powder on your skin or in your eyes when mixing the solution.** You may want to take the added precaution of wearing gloves and goggles. **Please see the "Important Safety Note" on page 13 for additional precautions regarding student use.**

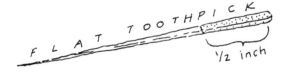

a. Make a "chemical scoop" out of a flat, wooden toothpick. Mark the toothpick one-half inch (about 1.25 cm) from its wide end. Use the area from the wide end of the toothpick to the mark to scoop up the indophenol powder. For the purposes of these instructions, consider "one scoop" to be as much powder as will fit on this area of the toothpick.

b. Make one gallon (3.8 liters) of indophenol solution by putting ten toothpick scoops (approximately 200 milligrams) of di-chloro-indophenol powder in a one-gallon (3.8 liter) container and filling the container to the top with tap water. Since the vitamin C titration used in this activity indicates relative amounts of vitamin C, the exact concentration of this indicator solution is unimportant.

c. Test the solution to see if it is approximately the right concentration: 4–8 drops of fresh or frozen orange juice should cause 10 ml of indophenol solution to lose all blue, violet, and pink tints. Make sure you stir the indophenol after the addition of each drop of juice. If the indophenol completes its color change after adding only 2–3 drops of juice, the solution is too dilute. Add another scoop of indophenol powder, mix thoroughly, and retest. If it takes more than 8 drops of juice to make the color change, the solution is too concentrated. Add more water and retest. This solution will remain stable for about a month.

Note: One gallon of indophenol solution is enough for a single class of 32 students to complete all the activities. If you have more than one class of students, or a very large number of liquids to test, it is best to mix all the indophenol solution you will need in one large container. That will ensure that the concentration of indophenol is the same for all tests, so the results of Session 1 can be compared to the results of Session 3. If you run out of indophenol and need to mix more, you can achieve nearly the same concentration by using the test described in step c. above. Or, if you have a chemical balance you can accurately measure 200 milligrams of indophenol for each gallon (3.8 liters) of water.

5. Fill the squeeze bottles labeled "Water" and "Indophenol Solution."

6. Make two copies of the data sheet for each student from the master on page 17. (Save the second copy for Session 3.)

7. (*Optional*) Make an overhead transparency of the data sheet. Using an overhead projector to demonstrate how to use the data sheet is very effective.

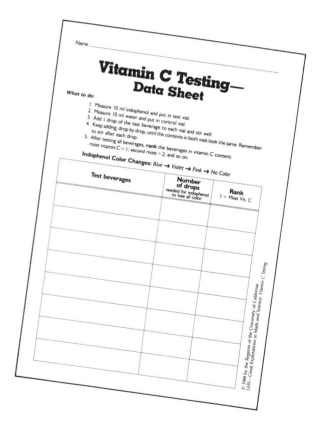

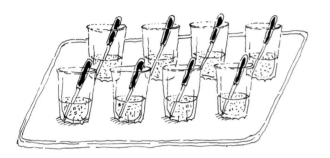

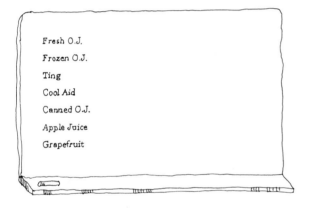

Fresh O.J.

Frozen O.J.

Ting

Cool Aid

Canned O.J.

Apple Juice

Grapefruit

The Day of the Activity:

1. If your students are testing fresh orange juice, squeeze enough to make two or three cups of juice. If the juice contains a lot of pulp that may clog the medicine droppers, you can put the juice into a blender and blend at medium speed for about 30 seconds. The blade will cut the pulp into tiny pieces, releasing the vitamin C contained in the pulp. If a blender is unavailable, you can strain the juice to remove the pulp. However, a fine-mesh strainer is likely to lower the vitamin C content, so avoid straining if possible.

2. Set out one tray for each group of 4–6 students. On each tray, place one cup with the name of each fruit drink. Fill all cups about one-third full and put a medicine dropper in each cup.

3. On a centrally located table, place: graduated cylinders, water bottles, bottles of indophenol, vials, stir sticks, white paper, and the data sheets. Also in this area should be a cup of vitamin C solution for each group of 4–6 students, about one-third full with a medicine dropper.

4. Arrange the room by pushing desks together or moving tables so that there is one flat work area for each group of 4–6 students. Place one large or several small fluid waste containers at each area.

5. List the names of the fruit beverages vertically on the board.

 Introducing the Procedure

1. Ask your students some questions about vitamin C: "Who has heard their parents or other adults talk about the importance of eating food that has vitamin C in it?" "What are some foods that contain vitamin C?" "Raise your hand if you take vitamin C tablets." "Why is vitamin C important to human health?"

These questions will allow your students to tell what they know about vitamin C, and start them wondering about its sources and uses. While you may want to mention some information about vitamin C at this point (see "Behind the Scenes," page 41), it is usually best to discuss background information **after** some of the hands-on activities.

2. Tell the class that today they will test various fruit drinks to see how much vitamin C the drinks contain. Point out the list of fruit drinks on the board and ask your students to predict which drink they think will contain the most vitamin C. Which do they predict will contain the least vitamin C? Tell them that you have also prepared some vitamin C solution. Explain how you prepared it and point out that it has more vitamin C in it than any of the fruit drinks.

3. Show the class a bottle of the indophenol solution (pronounced "in-dough-fin-all"). Tell them that this blue liquid is a vitamin C indicator—it can be used to indicate the amount of vitamin C in a liquid. Point out that indophenol solution is hazardous if swallowed.

Important Safety Note: Tell the students to avoid getting the indophenol solution on their skin. If they do, they should calmly walk to the sink and rinse it off with water. (If there is no sink in the classroom, they should use the water bottle to rinse their skin over a waste container). Caution the students against tasting any of the fruit drinks used in class because of the possibility that it might be contaminated with indophenol.

4. Demonstrate the test procedure to the class using fresh or frozen orange juice: (*Note:* Demonstrating the following procedure in front of a white background gives the students a better view of the color changes that occur. The demonstration can also be done on an overhead projector.)

> a. Measure 10 ml of indophenol solution and pour it into a vial. Set the vial on a sheet of white paper so it will be easier to make an accurate color determination. Explain that this is the "test vial."

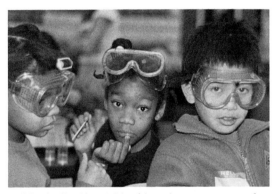

While the liquids used in this unit are not extremely hazardous, having students wear safety goggles establishes good laboratory safety practice. Class sets of safety goggles can be borrowed from high school science labs.

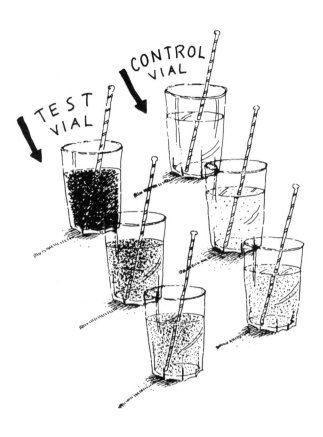

b. Measure 10 ml of water and pour it into a second vial. Set this vial next to the test vial on the white paper. Tell the students that this vial is the "control vial."

c. Use a medicine dropper to add one drop of orange juice to the test vial and one drop of orange juice to the control vial. After the addition of each drop stir thoroughly, using a separate stir stick for each vial. Continue adding drops of orange juice, first to the test vial and then to the control vial, remembering to stir after each drop. Have your students count the number of drops you add to each vial.

d. Tell your students that the goal of this test is to count how many drops of orange juice are required to cause the contents of the test vial to become the same color as the contents of the control vial. As a liquid with vitamin C is added, the indophenol will change from blue→violet→pink→no color. When the indophenol loses its color, the contents of the two vials will become the same color. This is called the *end point*. Ask your students to tell you when the contents of the two vials look similar. If there are any doubts, add another drop to see if the color changes.

e. When the end point has been reached, hold up the two vials and ask if they are totally clear. [No, they will have an orange tint.] Point out that if the juice is colored, there will always be a tint to the solution, even when the indophenol becomes colorless. This is why the control vial is used. When the color of the contents of the two vials is the same, they will know that all color due to the indophenol is gone.

f. Demonstrate how to dump out the contents of the vials into a waste container, and use a water bottle to rinse the vials and stir sticks with water. Ask your students what might happen if they don't rinse their equipment between each test. [The vials will be contaminated, so the test results will be inaccurate.]

5. Explain how to use the data sheet. If you are using an overhead projector, demonstrate using a transparency. Otherwise, hold up a data sheet. Show your students how to write the name of a fruit drink in the first column and record the number of drops required to titrate it in the second column. If it takes more than 50 drops to reach the end point, students should record "50+." Mention that when they finish testing all of the fruit drinks they will rank the beverages from most vitamin C (#1) to least vitamin C, and write the rank in the third column.

6. Tell the class that the procedure of adding one liquid to another drop by drop until a specified end point is reached is called a *titration.* Write the word *titration* on the board.

Explaining How a Titration Indicates Vitamin C Content

1. Ask a representative from each pair of students to come to the equipment table and get two data sheets and one of each piece of equipment.

2. Give one cup of vitamin C solution to each group. Do not distribute the trays of fruit drinks yet. Have students work in pairs, using vitamin C solution to titrate the indophenol in the test vial and the water in the control vial.

3. When all teams have completed this test, focus the attention of the entire class. Ask:

- How many drops did it take to titrate the indophenol with vitamin C solution? [1–2 drops.]

- How many drops did it take to titrate the indophenol with orange juice in the demonstration? [4–8 drops.]

- How many drops do you predict something with very little vitamin C would take to titrate the indophenol? [A lot of drops.]

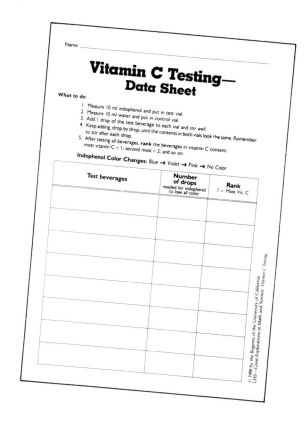

Name _____

Vitamin C Testing—
Data Sheet

What to do:

1. Measure 10 ml indophenol and put in test vial.
2. Measure 10 ml water and put in control vial.
3. Add 1 drop of the test beverage to each vial and stir well.
4. Keep adding, drop by drop, until the contents in both vials look the same. Remember to stir after each drop.
5. After testing all beverages, **rank** the beverages in vitamin C content: most vitamin C = 1; second most = 2; and so on.

Indophenol Color Changes: Blue → Violet → Pink → No Color

Test beverages	Number of drops needed for indophenol to lose all color	Rank 1 = Most Vit. C

© 1988 by the Regents of the University of California
LHS—Great Explorations in Math and Science: *Vitamin C Testing*

4. Explain that vitamin C reacts with the indophenol and causes its color to change. A liquid containing a lot of vitamin C needs just one drop to cause all of the indophenol to react. Many drops of a liquid containing only a small amount of vitamin C must be added to cause all of the indophenol to react.

5. Summarize the relationship this way: the **fewer** drops required to titrate indophenol, the **greater** the amount of vitamin C contained in the liquid. This inverse relation may seem confusing at first, since we don't usually expect that the less you add of one thing, the more of something else is present. Your students may not understand this right away. It will be reinforced later in this activity and again in Session 2.

Testing the Beverages

1. Distribute one tray of beverages to each group of students. Have pairs of students work together to test all of the fruit beverages.

2. As teams finish, instruct them to rank the juices based on their results, with "#1" indicating the greatest concentration of vitamin C. They should write these ranking numbers in the last column of their data sheets.

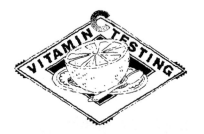

Name _____

Vitamin C Testing— Data Sheet

What to do:

1. Measure 10 ml indophenol and put in test vial.
2. Measure 10 ml water and put in control vial.
3. Add 1 drop of the test beverage to each vial and *stir well.*
4. Keep adding, drop by drop, until the contents in both vials look the same. Remember to stir after each drop.
5. After testing all beverages, **rank** the beverages in vitamin C content: most vitamin C = 1; second most = 2; and so on.

Indophenol Color Changes: *Blue* → *Violet* → *Pink* → *No Color*

Test beverages	Number of drops needed for indophenol to lose all color	Rank 1 = Most Vit. C

LHS—Great Explorations in Math and Science: *Vitamin C Testing*

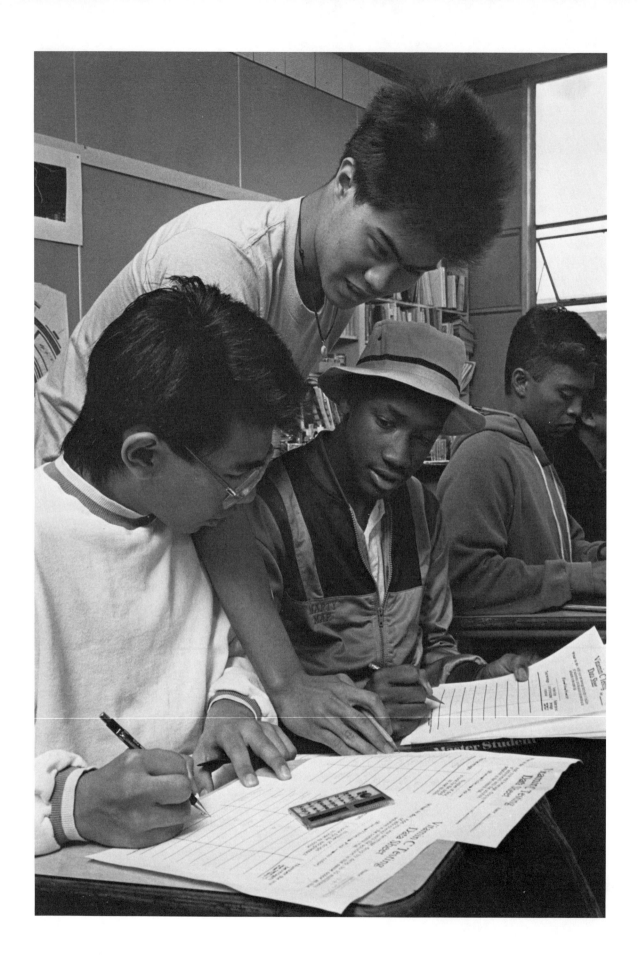

Session 2: Analyzing the Results

Overview

In this session, the students pool data from Session 1, calculate averages, and construct a bar graph. They then draw conclusions about the relative amounts of vitamin C in each drink, and which food processes (such as fresh squeezing, freezing, or canning) are better for preserving vitamin C content.

The purpose of this session is for the students to develop skills in analyzing and interpreting data. They are also provided with scientific and nutritional information on vitamin C.

What You Need

For the class:
- ☐ chalkboard and chalk
- ☐ 1 or more calculators or scratch paper and pencils
- ☐ (*Optional*) overhead projector and blank transparency

For each pair of students:
- ☐ completed data sheets from Session 1
- ☐ 2 graphing sheets (master included on page 23)
- ☐ colored pencils (or crayons or colored pens)

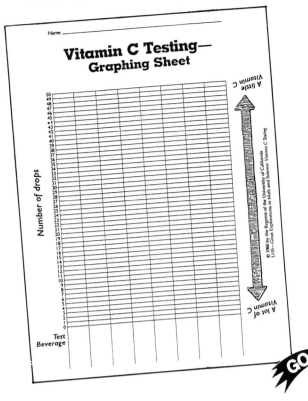

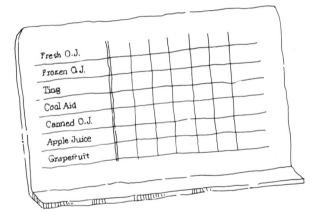

Getting Ready

1. Make one copy of the graphing sheet for each student, from the master on page 23.

2. (*Optional*) If you will be using an overhead projector, make a transparency of the graphing sheet.

3. Write the name of each drink that was tested in a vertical list on the left side of the chalkboard. Draw a grid to the right to record the results of each team.

Pooling the Data

1. Have one member from each team report how many drops of the first drink listed on the board were needed to titrate the indophenol. Record each group's data next to the name of that drink. Repeat this procedure to collect data for all of the fruit drinks.

2. When you have collected all of the data, ask your students how it is that different teams, conducting the same test on the same item, can get different results. Accept their suggestions for sources of error. Ask what they think scientists do when they don't agree on experimental results. [Repeat the tests, see how testing procedures might have differed, average the results.] Tell them that today they'll be averaging their results.

3. If your students know how to calculate averages, assign pairs of students to calculate the averages of one or two test items. Distribute calculators (if they're available) or have students calculate using pencil and paper to find the average number of drops it took to titrate the fruit drinks. If your students are not familiar with averages and how to calculate them, take this opportunity to introduce the concept and the procedure, and let them use this exercise as practice.

4. Record the average values for each fruit drink on the board.

Making Bar Graphs

1. When all of the averages have been calculated, show the students how to make bar graphs using the graphing sheet.

2. Demonstrate how to make a bar graph by writing the name of the first drink at the base of the first column and coloring in the column up to the average number of drops required to titrate with that drink. Explain that later you will show them how to use the upside-down writing on the right. Distribute one graphing sheet to each student and have your students make bar graphs with all of the average values.

3. When most of your students have finished, focus the attention of the entire class. Ask your students if the tallest bars on their graph represent those juices containing the most vitamin C. [No. Those drinks have the least vitamin C.]

4. Tell the students to turn their graphs upside down so the words "A Lot of Vitamin C" and "A Little Vitamin C" are right-side-up on the left side of the paper. Ask them to imagine that the uncolored part of the column is a bar representing the amount of vitamin C contained in each beverage. To make this more apparent, you could have your students color in these "blank" bars.

5. Ask the class to tell you the name of the beverage with the most vitamin C, the juice with the second most vitamin C content, and so on. As the group ranks the juices, record the ranking by writing numbers next to the name of each beverage on the board—#1, #2, etc.

6. If some students have not understood the inverse relation between the number of drops required to titrate indophenol and the vitamin C content, discuss and clarify this by reminding the students how many drops were needed for the vitamin C solution [only 1 or 2 drops].

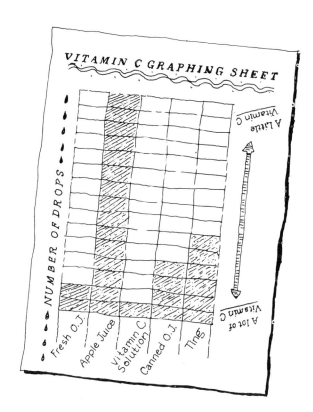

Drawing Conclusions

1. Discuss what conclusions can be drawn from the results: Which juice would you drink if you wanted the most vitamin C? Which drink would you avoid if you wanted the most vitamin C? Point out that some of these juices may have had vitamin C added to them and others contain naturally-occurring vitamin C.

2. Spend five to ten minutes giving your students information about vitamin C. Refer to "Behind the Scenes" on page 41 for a brief summary of: the role of vitamin C in our bodies; which parts of which plants are the best sources of vitamin C; the discovery of the need for vitamin C; and the range of recommended daily allowances of vitamin C.

3. Tell the class that you would like them to bring in fruit drinks from home for the next session, to see how much vitamin C they contain. **Tell them not to bring in red and purple colored juices because their color masks indophenol's color changes.**

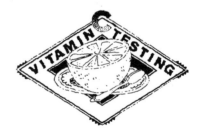

Name _____

Vitamin C Testing— Graphing Sheet

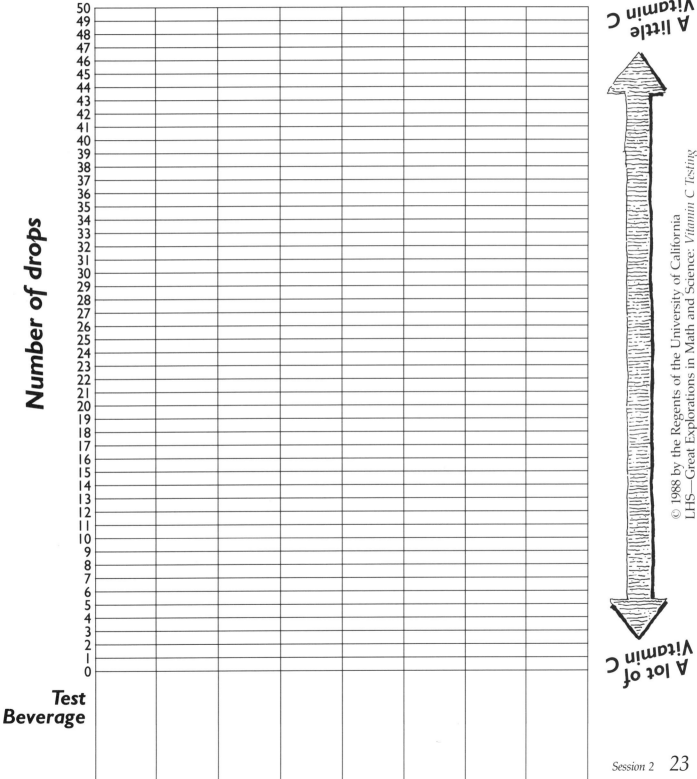

Number of drops

50
49
48
47
46
45
44
43
42
41
40
39
38
37
36
35
34
33
32
31
30
29
28
27
26
25
24
23
22
21
20
19
18
17
16
15
14
13
12
11
10
9
8
7
6
5
4
3
2
1
0

Test Beverage

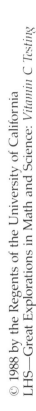

A little Vitamin C

A lot of Vitamin C

© 1988 by the Regents of the University of California
LHS—Great Explorations in Math and Science: *Vitamin C Testing*

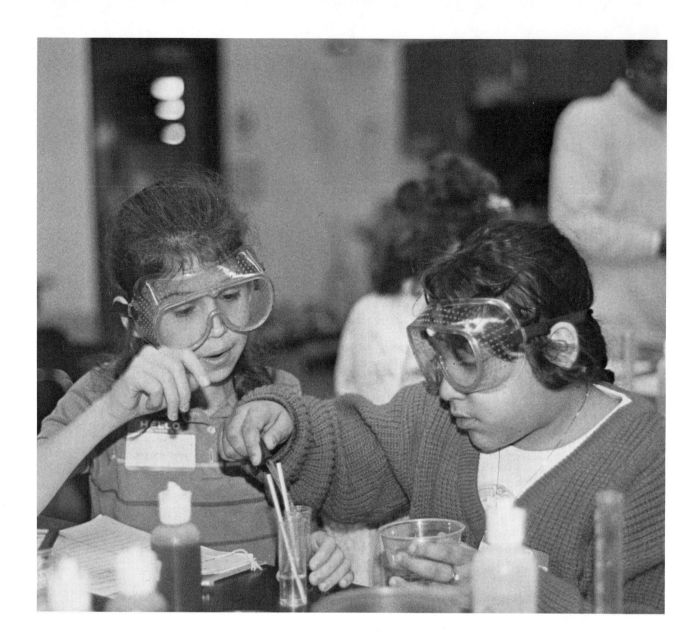

Session 3: Testing More Beverages

Overview

Now that your students are familiar with a method of testing for vitamin C, they can use it to determine the relative vitamin C content of beverages they drink at home. One of the strongest aspects of this activity is that it connects what students have learned to their daily diet. Also, testing beverages from home commonly draws parents, brothers, and sisters into the action. Your students will assume the role of experts when they are asked by family members about the results of their tests.

While this session provides further practice in laboratory techniques, and in analyzing and interpreting data, the primary objective is for the students to apply what they learn to their own diets. For this reason, it is important that they test liquids they actually drink at home. Since many students forget to bring in things from home, it is advisable to plan this unit a few days in advance, and to keep reminding your students to bring the juices to school.

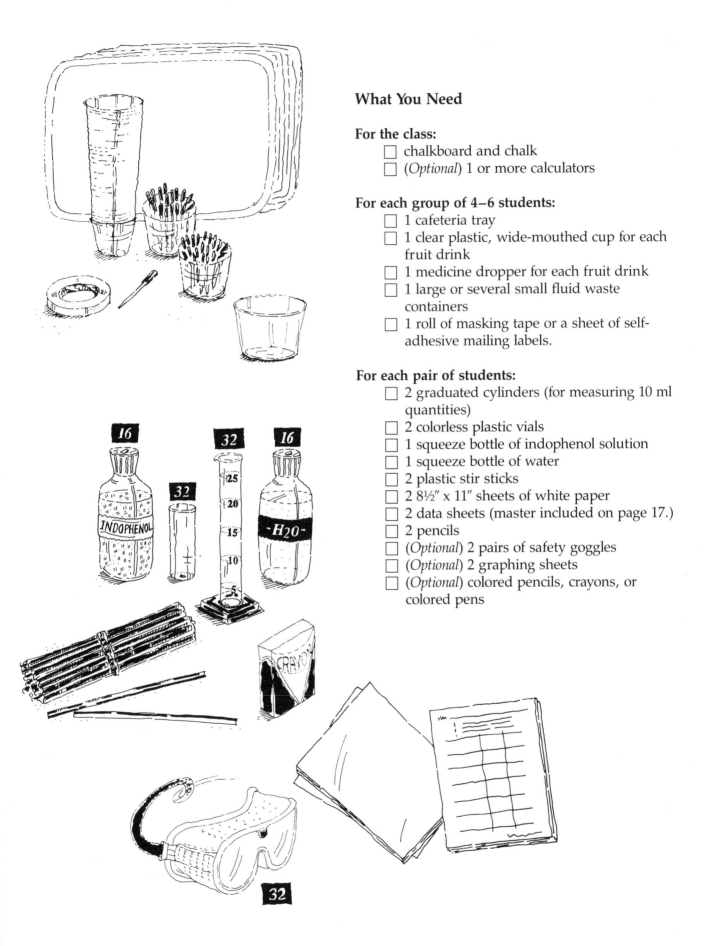

What You Need

For the class:
- ☐ chalkboard and chalk
- ☐ (*Optional*) 1 or more calculators

For each group of 4–6 students:
- ☐ 1 cafeteria tray
- ☐ 1 clear plastic, wide-mouthed cup for each fruit drink
- ☐ 1 medicine dropper for each fruit drink
- ☐ 1 large or several small fluid waste containers
- ☐ 1 roll of masking tape or a sheet of self-adhesive mailing labels.

For each pair of students:
- ☐ 2 graduated cylinders (for measuring 10 ml quantities)
- ☐ 2 colorless plastic vials
- ☐ 1 squeeze bottle of indophenol solution
- ☐ 1 squeeze bottle of water
- ☐ 2 plastic stir sticks
- ☐ 2 8½" x 11" sheets of white paper
- ☐ 2 data sheets (master included on page 17.)
- ☐ 2 pencils
- ☐ (*Optional*) 2 pairs of safety goggles
- ☐ (*Optional*) 2 graphing sheets
- ☐ (*Optional*) colored pencils, crayons, or colored pens

Getting Ready

Before the Day of the Activity:

1. Remind your students to bring in fruit beverages from home.

2. Check to see that materials used in Session 1 are ready for use:

  a. Prepare more indophenol solution if necessary. (See Session 1, "Getting Ready Before the Day of the Activity," page 10 for instructions.)

  b. Refill the squeeze bottles labeled "Water" and "Indophenol Solution."

  c. Duplicate more data sheets if necessary, using the master on page 17.

  d. (*Optional*) If you want your students to graph the results, duplicate graphing sheets using the master on page 23.

The Day of the Activity:

1. Set out one tray for each group of 4–6 students. On each tray, place 4–6 cups, 4–6 medicine droppers, and some masking tape. The students from each group will use this equipment and the beverages they have brought from home to prepare labeled cups of each new fruit drink.

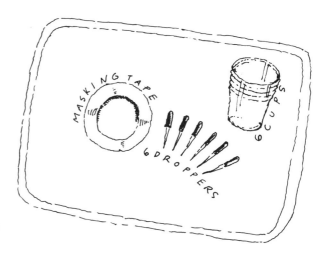

2. On a centrally located table, place: graduated cylinders, water bottles, bottles of indophenol, vials, stir sticks, white paper, and the data sheets.

3. Arrange the room by pushing desks together or moving tables so that there is one flat work area for each group of 4–6 students. Place one large or several small fluid waste containers at each area.

Conducting the Tests

1. Have your students place the fruit drinks they brought from home on their group's tray. If some groups have brought in fewer drinks, you might want to redistribute the test items so every group has about the same number.

2. Instruct each group of 4–6 students to use the masking tape and a pencil to label one cup with the name of each test item. Have them fill the labeled cups about one-third full with their fruit drinks and place a medicine dropper in each cup.

3. Ask a representative from each pair of students to come to the equipment table and get two data sheets and one of each piece of equipment.

4. Have pairs of students work together to test each fruit drink at their table. Each fruit drink will therefore be tested by 4–6 students.

Drawing Conclusions

1. As your students finish, have them place all cups and medicine droppers back on the trays and place the trays and all other equipment on the equipment table. Distribute calculators (if available) and have each group of 4–6 students calculate, for each test item, the average number of drops required to titrate the indophenol solution.

2. Have a member from each group write the averages on the board. Organize the results by having each group write their results under one of the following headings: fresh juices, frozen juices, canned juices, juices made from powders, etc. Or, rather than listing the juices by storage method, they could be listed by type of fruit: orange, grapefruit, lemon, apple, etc. Organizing the results often allows patterns to be seen more easily.

3. Lead a class discussion of the results: "Which results are surprising to you?" "Do you notice any patterns in the results?" "Do our results indicate that canned fruit drinks have less vitamin C than fresh juices?" and so on.

4. Ask if anyone can think of a reason why one orange juice might have a different amount of vitamin C than another orange juice. [Some orange juices are diluted with water; some drinks use artificial orange flavor and sugar; some orange juices are heated or frozen before packaging; some orange juices may have been on the shelf longer than others; different orange juices are made from oranges grown in regions with varying weather and soil conditions.]

5. Ask your students if they think it's fair to assume that two juices with the same vitamin C content are equally good from a nutritional standpoint. [Not necessarily. Juices contain more than just vitamin C. The presence of other vitamins, added sugar, sugar substitutes, or artificial additives are all factors to consider.]

6. There is usually not enough time for your students to create bar graphs of this data. If you want your students to have a chance to do this, have someone copy the data from the board. Duplicate this data and distribute it with a graphing sheet for each student to do as a homework assignment. Alternatively, the data can be used by the group to create a large bar graph on butcher paper to post on the wall. If you decide to do this, plan an extra class session.

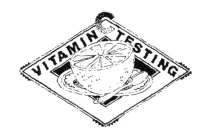

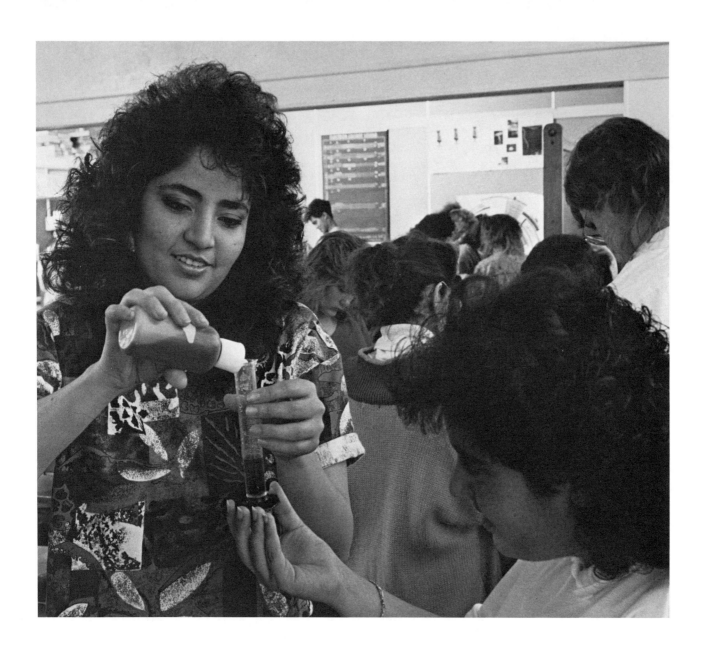

Session 4: Experimenting with Vitamin C Content

Overview

In this session, your students conduct one or more experiments comparing two different treatments of the same juice to determine the effects on vitamin C content. The first experiment is suggested by the question, "What happens if you forget to put the lid back on the bottle of juice and leave it out overnight?" You may also decide to have your students experiment with the effects of boiling and freezing.

The equipment used in this activity is not as sensitive as professional lab equipment, so your students may not always obtain expected results. The various lab teams may even come to different conclusions. In such cases it is often helpful to look at the pattern of data from the entire class, to discuss what might have caused the differences, and to average results.

The primary objective is for the students to develop skills in conducting experiments and interpreting data. Possible misconceptions about the effects of specific food processing methods can be corrected at the end of the activity by relating the conclusions of scientists who have studied these same questions with more accurate equipment.

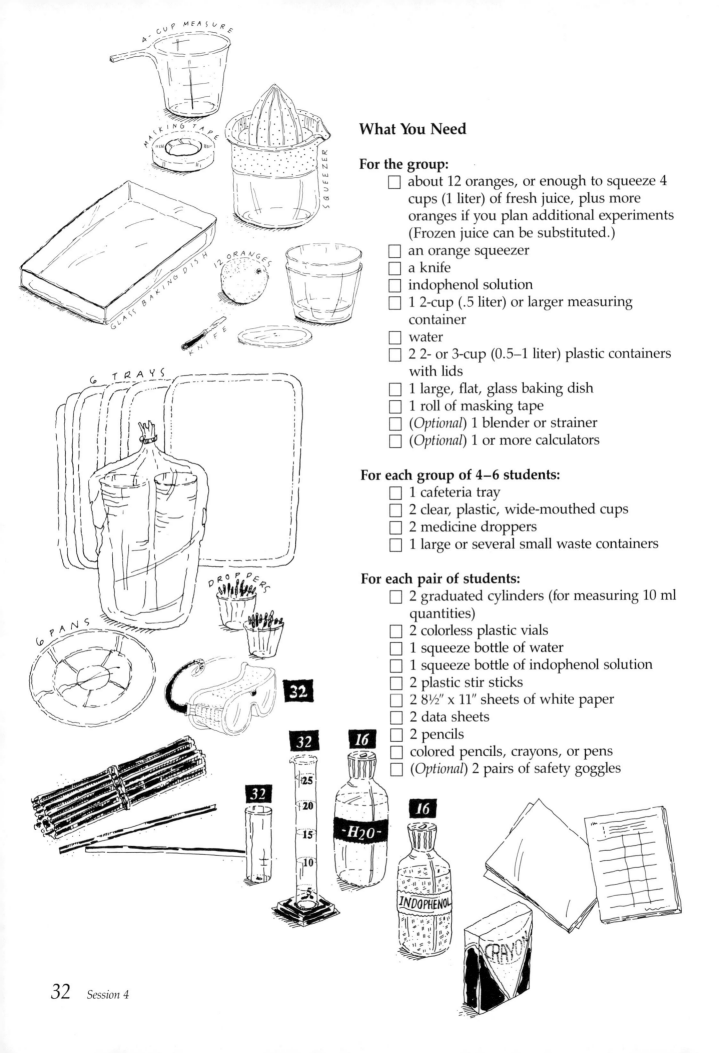

What You Need

For the group:
- [ ] about 12 oranges, or enough to squeeze 4 cups (1 liter) of fresh juice, plus more oranges if you plan additional experiments (Frozen juice can be substituted.)
- [ ] an orange squeezer
- [ ] a knife
- [ ] indophenol solution
- [ ] 1 2-cup (.5 liter) or larger measuring container
- [ ] water
- [ ] 2 2- or 3-cup (0.5–1 liter) plastic containers with lids
- [ ] 1 large, flat, glass baking dish
- [ ] 1 roll of masking tape
- [ ] (*Optional*) 1 blender or strainer
- [ ] (*Optional*) 1 or more calculators

For each group of 4–6 students:
- [ ] 1 cafeteria tray
- [ ] 2 clear, plastic, wide-mouthed cups
- [ ] 2 medicine droppers
- [ ] 1 large or several small waste containers

For each pair of students:
- [ ] 2 graduated cylinders (for measuring 10 ml quantities)
- [ ] 2 colorless plastic vials
- [ ] 1 squeeze bottle of water
- [ ] 1 squeeze bottle of indophenol solution
- [ ] 2 plastic stir sticks
- [ ] 2 8½" x 11" sheets of white paper
- [ ] 2 data sheets
- [ ] 2 pencils
- [ ] colored pencils, crayons, or pens
- [ ] (*Optional*) 2 pairs of safety goggles

Getting Ready

You will need to begin preparation two days prior to this session. With more mature groups, involving the students in planning and preparing the experiment is highly recommended.

Two Days Before the Activity:

1. Squeeze enough oranges to make four cups of juice. If the juice contains a lot of pulp that may clog the medicine droppers, you can put the juice into a blender and blend at medium speed for about 30 seconds. The blade will cut the pulp into tiny pieces releasing the vitamin C contained in the pulp. If a blender is unavailable, you may strain the juice to remove the pulp. However, a fine-mesh strainer is likely to lower the vitamin C content, so avoid straining if possible.

2. Divide the total amount of orange juice into two equal amounts, and perform the following treatments:

   a. **Left out, uncovered:** Pour the two cups of orange juice into a large rectangular baking dish. Leave it in the room, uncovered for 48 hours. (A large, flat, baking dish is used to increase the amount of orange juice exposed to the air.) After two days, pour the juice into a measuring container and add water so the total volume is equal to its initial volume—two cups. (Replacing the evaporated water turns out to be important to make sure that the variable of concentration is controlled.)

   b. **Covered and put in refrigerator:** Put the remaining two cups of orange juice in a covered container in the refrigerator for two days prior to conducting the activity. This juice will be compared to the juice that was left out in the room, exposed to air.

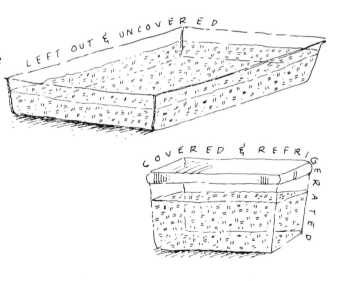

Note: Comparing these two treatments will maximize the observable difference caused by two variables that often occur together in real life: forgetting to put the juice in the refrigerator and exposing it to the air. While it is not realistic to spread out the juice in a baking dish, doing so increases the chance that your students will observe a reduction in vitamin C. Scientists often perform such experiments to see if there is an effect worth further investigation. Advanced students may wish to separate the effects of these variables through further experiments.

3. (*Optional*) If you wish to extend the experiments to investigating the effects of freezing and boiling, decide on the most appropriate method for your group of students. Younger students should first complete the investigation described above. They should then repeat the experiment, starting with more fresh juice, this time comparing boiled or frozen juice with untreated juice. Older students may do all of these experiments at once with eight cups of juice: Keep two cups in a closed container in the refrigerator, treat two cups by exposure to air as described above, freeze two cups and boil two cups. Freezing and boiling treatments are described below:

    c. **Frozen:** Pour the orange juice in a plastic container with a lid and freeze it. Start thawing it out the day before class.

    d. **Boiled:** Pour the orange juice into a non-aluminum saucepan and boil it for 20 minutes. Pour the boiled juice into a measuring container and add water so the total volume is equal to its initial volume. Cool the juice and put it in a covered container in the refrigerator.

Note: The following instructions assume you are conducting only the simpler experiment (which compares juice that is left at room temperature and exposed to air with juice that is covered and kept in the refrigerator). You should adapt the experiment to include the other treatments if you decide to conduct them.

The Day Before the Activity:

1. Use masking tape to label plastic cups to say: "O.J.—Left Out," and "O.J.—Covered & Refrigerated." You'll need to label one set of these cups for each group of 4–6 students.

2. Check to see that materials used in Session 1 are ready for use:

    a. Prepare more indophenol solution if necessary. (See Session 1, "Getting Ready, Before the Day of the Activity," page 10 for instructions.)

    b. Refill the squeeze bottles labeled "Water" and "Indophenol Solution."

    c. Duplicate more data sheets if necessary, using the master on page 17.

The Day of the Activity:

1. Set out one tray for each group of 4–6 students. On each tray, place one set of the cups you labeled for this session. Fill all cups about one third full and put one medicine dropper in each cup.

2. On a centrally located table, place: graduated cylinders, water bottles, bottles of indophenol, vials, stir sticks, white paper, and the data sheets.

3. Arrange the room as you did in Session 1: pushing desks together or moving tables so that there is one flat work area for each group of 4–6 students. Place one large or several small waste containers at each area.

4. List the treated juices on the left side of the chalkboard. Draw a grid to the right to record the results of each team.

Experimenting

1. Ask the students for their opinions about why parents sometimes remind their children to "Cover the juice and put it away in the refrigerator." [Expect a variety of answers, such as "It keeps the juice from spoiling," or "To keep it cold."] If the students do not think of it, ask if they think the vitamin C content may be affected if the juice is left out of the refrigerator all night. Tell them that they will do an experiment to find out if vitamin C content is affected by leaving juice unrefrigerated and exposed to the air for two days.

2. Describe exactly how you treated the juice that was left out and explain how you treated the juice that was covered and refrigerated. Emphasize that both juices were prepared from the same batch of oranges, so they started out with the same vitamin C content. Ask the students to predict which juice (if any) might have less vitamin C.

3. Have one representative from each pair of students come to the equipment table and get two data sheets and one of each piece of equipment.

4. Distribute one tray of juices to each station and have students work in pairs to test them.

5. When the students finish testing the different juice samples, collect the trays of juices and equipment.

Pooling Data and Analyzing Results

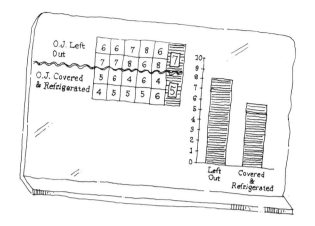

1. As teams finish their tests, have them write their results on the chalkboard next to the description of each treated juice.

2. Assign individuals to calculate class averages for each treated juice.

3. Make a bar graph on the chalkboard, where the vertical axis goes in increments of 1 drop and ranges from 0–10 drops. When all of the averages have been calculated, ask two student volunteers to come up and make a bar representing the results of each treatment group.

4. Ask the class what conclusions can be drawn from the results. Based on these results, can we conclude that there is a nutritional basis for covering bottles of juice and putting them in the refrigerator? Explain to the class that other scientists have found that exposure to air does destroy vitamin C.

5. Sometimes the students' results may be unclear, or contradict what other scientists have found. If this occurs, ask the class to think of reasons that could explain why their results might be different. [e.g., "Maybe their orange juice was exposed to the air longer than ours."] **It is important that students do not feel like they got the "wrong answer," but rather understand that there are logical reasons why scientists sometimes get conflicting results.** Ask the students if they can think of a better way to set up this experiment.

6. Spend a few minutes providing students with information about loss and retention of vitamins in food preparation and storage. (See "Behind the Scenes," page 41 for information.)

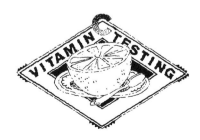

Going Further

1. Use the packaging from the fruit drinks your students tested to conduct an investigation of product labeling. Discuss advertising claims that appear on the packaging. Which beverages have naturally-occurring vitamin C and which ones have vitamin C added to them? Introduce the concept of minimum daily requirement. How much of each beverage would be needed to meet the minimum daily requirement of vitamin C? What other ingredients are added to the juices?

2. Have the class conduct a study of vitamin C content in oranges over time. Buy six oranges and store them in the classroom. Have your students test the vitamin C content of one orange per week to investigate whether old oranges have less vitamin C than fresh oranges.

3. When potatoes are cut into slices and left out in the air they turn brown. But if they are coated with lemon juice, they keep their natural color. Is this due to the vitamin C content of lemon juice? The acid content of the juice? Or to something else? Have your class investigate this phenomenon by cutting several slices of potatoes and painting half of each slice with these liquids: concentrated vitamin C solution, lemon juice, orange juice, and vinegar. The first three liquids contain various amounts of vitamin C. Vinegar contains acetic acid, but no vitamin C (ascorbic acid). Check the slices after 15 minutes, 1 hour, 3 hours, and 24 hours. What can your students conclude from their experiment? Try the experiment with other fruits and vegetables that turn brown (bananas and apples) and other liquids (apple juice, grapefruit juice, coffee, etc.)

4. The indophenol titration provides information about *relative* vitamin C content. Advanced students can figure out *absolute* vitamin C content by calibrating the titration. This is done by creating solutions of vitamin C of different concentrations, testing each solution to see how many drops are required to titrate the indophenol, and then graphing these results. After calibrating the titration, you can find the absolute vitamin C concentration of any beverage by titrating it and then looking on the graph to see the corresponding amount of vitamin C.

The ratios and proportions involved in making solutions of different concentrations are difficult for students to understand. Consequently, it is best if you set up the successive dilutions and label containers of vitamin C solutions with the appropriate concentration. Here's how to prepare the solutions:

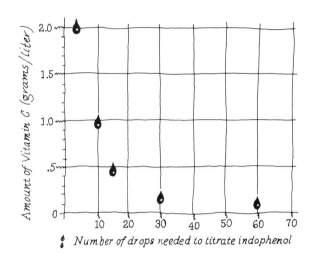

Number of drops needed to titrate indophenol

a. Dissolve 1 500-mg tablet of vitamin C in 250 ml of water. This is a 500 mg/250 ml or 2 g/liter solution.

b. Measure 125 ml of the 2 g/liter vitamin C solution and pour it in a 250 ml container. Add water to make 250 ml. This is a 250 mg/250 ml or 1g/liter solution.

c. Measure 125 ml of the 1 g/liter vitamin C solution and pour it in a 250 ml container. Add water to make 250 ml. This is a 125 mg/250 ml or 0.5g/liter solution.

d. Measure 100 ml of the 0.5 g/liter vitamin C solution and pour it in a 250 ml container. Add water to make 250 ml. This is a 50 mg/250 ml or 0.2g/liter solution.

e. Measure 125 ml of the 0.2 g/liter vitamin C solution and pour it in a 250 ml container. Add water to make 250 ml. This is a 25 mg/250 ml or 0.1 g/liter solution.

Have your students determine how much of each one of these vitamin C solutions is required to titrate 10 ml of indophenol. Then make a graph of concentration vs. number of drops required to titrate 10 ml of indophenol. This graph can be used to convert relative vitamin C content (expressed in number of drops required to titrate the indophenol) to absolute concentration of vitamin C in fruit beverages.

5. The GEMS unit entitled *Paper Towel Testing* is an excellent follow-up to this unit. It is also concerned with consumer science, but allows the students greater latitude in designing their own experiments.

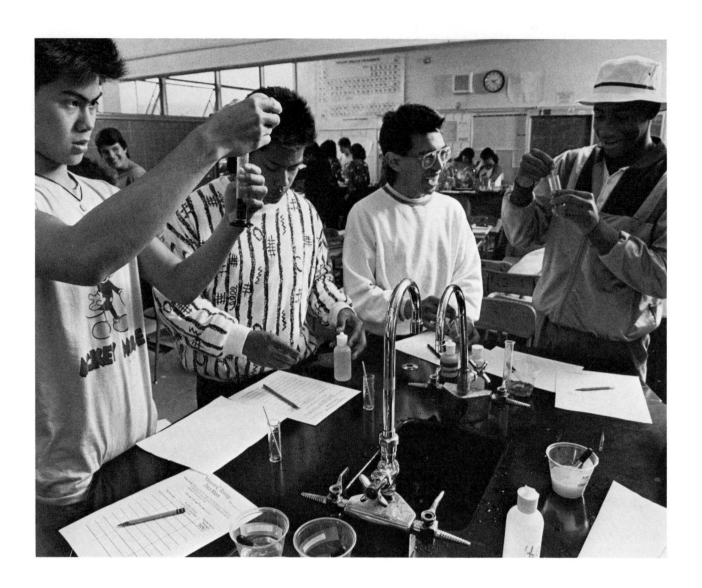

Behind the Scenes

The following information on vitamin C is included to assist the teacher in providing students with some additional background. **It is not meant to be read out loud to the class, but to be communicated by the teacher at whatever level is appropriate.**

Vitamin C is very important to human health. While research continues on all the ways that vitamin C contributes to our bodies, it is known that it helps in the formation of connective tissue, bone, teeth, and blood vessel walls, and assists the body in assimilating other important substances, such as iron and some amino acids.

Serious deficiencies of vitamin C harm the entire body. Scurvy is the name of the disease caused by such deficiency, and sailors on long voyages often suffered from scurvy. Then it was discovered that eating citrus fruits would prevent the disease. Large sailing expeditions began bringing crates of limes on long voyages, accounting for the origin of the old nickname for British sailors—"Limeys." When the limes were no longer available, sailors were able to augment their vitamin C intake by eating large quantities of potatoes. Scientists recognized that limes (and to a lesser extent potatoes) contained a substance that prevented scurvy, and they named this substance "vitamin C."

Many years later, in 1937, Dr. Albert Szent-Gyorgyi won a Nobel prize for isolating vitamin C. He began his research to find out why bananas and apples turn brown when exposed to air, while other foods, such as citrus fruits, do not. He discovered that vitamin C, the anti-scurvy vitamin, was responsible for keeping fruits from turning brown. That is why putting lemon juice on apples and bananas after they are peeled or sliced helps them keep their natural color.

Although vitamin C is found in many plants, and is synthesized by many animals, humans do not create their own, and must consume it in foods. Plants manufacture vitamin C during the process of photosynthesis. The more light a plant gets, the more photosynthetic activity, and the more vitamin C produced. More light also results in darker-colored leaves, and it's generally true that the darker the leaf, the more vitamin C the plant contains.

Among fruits high in vitamin C are all citrus fruits, strawberries, and pineapples. Citrus *peels* contain five to seven times *more* vitamin C than does the juice. Vegetables with particularly high vitamin C content include sweet peppers, cabbage, brussels sprouts, broccoli, and spinach.

Opinions differ regarding the recommended daily requirement for vitamin C in human nutrition. It has been established that 10 mg of vitamin C per day will prevent scurvy. In the United States, the recommended daily allowance (RDA) of vitamin C is 60 mg per day, but it is 30 mg in Norway and Canada, and 70 mg in West Germany. The famous scientist Linus Pauling advocates that people take as much as 3,000 mg per day. One cup of fresh orange juice provides about 125 mg of vitamin C.

Because vitamin C is a water-soluble vitamin (as is vitamin B) it is easily leached out of fruits and vegetables in boiling water. It is also sensitive to heat and light and can be lost through exposure to air, certain metals, and some enzymes, but it is not lost by freezing. Because it is water soluble, when vitamin C reaches an excessive level in the body it is excreted in the urine. There are also fat-soluble vitamins, such as vitamins A, D, E, and K, which tend not to leach out in boiling water. These vitamins can accumulate in the fatty tissues of our bodies if taken in excessive amounts. In some cases, the storage and concentration of these fat-soluble vitamins in the body can be a health hazard.

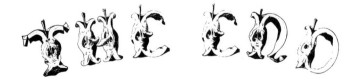

Resources

Indophenol Powder

2, 6, di-chloro-indophenol, sodium salt is an indicator for ascorbic acid (vitimin C). When dissolved in water, it forms a blue solution. Ascorbic acid reduces indophenol solution to a colorless liquid. A 1 gram quantity of indophenol powder will be enough to present this unit several times. It can be purchased inexpensively from:

> Flinn Scientific, Inc.
> P.O. Box 219
> 131 Flinn St.
> Batavia, IL 60510
> (708) 879-6900

Plastic vials

Colorless plastic vials with a 30–40 ml (7–10 dram) capacity can be purchased inexpensively from:

> **Nasco**
> 901 Janesville Ave.
> Fort Atkinson, WI 53538
> (800) 558-9595
> (referred to as Drosophilia Culture Vials)

> **Sargent-Welch Scientific Company**
> 7300 North Linder Ave.
> P.O. Box 1026
> Skokie, IL 60077
> (800) 422-4280

> **VWR Scientific**
> 3745 Bayshore Blvd.
> Brisbane, CA 94005
> (415) 468-7150

Summary Outlines

Session 1: Conducting the Tests

Getting Ready
Before the Day of the Activity:
1. Purchase fruit juices
2. Assemble materials.
3. Label containers.
4. Prepare test juices.
5. Prepare indophenol solution.
6. Fill squeeze bottles with water and indophenol solution.
7. Duplicate data sheets.
8. (*Optional*) Make overhead transparency of data sheet.

The Day of the Activity:
1. Squeeze and blend orange juice.
2. Pour drinks into cups, add medicine droppers, set on trays.
3. Place cups of vitamin C and all other equipment on centrally located table.
4. Arrange room in work stations for groups of 4–6 students.
5. Write the names of the fruit drinks vertically on board.

Introducing the Procedure
1. Ask students what they know about vitamin C.
2. Explain challenge: to test fruit drinks for vitamin C.
3. List drinks you have prepared.
4. Ask students for predictions.
5. Discuss indophenol, and concept of indicator.
6. Mention safety precautions.
7. Demonstrate procedure:
   a. Measure 10 ml indophenol—test vial.
   b. Measure 10 ml water—control vial.
   c. Add orange juice to each vial, drop-by-drop, stirring thoroughly after each drop.
   d. Count drops until contents of vials look the same. This is the **end point.**
   f. Compare both vials. Explain reason for control vial.
   g. Demonstrate how to rinse equipment.
8. Show how to record data.
9. Introduce concept of **titration.**

Explaining How a Titration Indicates Vitamin C
Content
1. Pairs of students get equipment and data sheets.
2. Distribute vitamin C solution.
3. Students test vitamin C solution and compare
   with results of orange juice.
4. Explain that the fewer drops required to titrate,
   the more vitamin C.

Testing the Juices
1. Distribute trays of juices.
2. Have teams test juices.
3. Have teams rank juices according to amount of
   vitamin C.

Session 2: Analyzing the Results

Getting Ready
1. Duplicate graphing sheets
2. Write names of fruit drinks on board
3. (*Optional*) Make overhead transparency of data
   sheet.

Pooling the Data
1. Teams report data.
2. Ask why different students get different results.
3. Explain technique of averaging (if necessary).
4. Distribute calculators and have students average
   results.
5. Record average values on board.

Making Bar Graphs
1. Demonstrate how to make bar graphs.
2. Distribute graphing sheets.
3. Have each student make bar graph of results.
4. Explain inverse relation between drops and
   vitamin C.
5. As a group, rank the results.

Drawing Conclusions
1. Ask what conclusions can be drawn.
2. Give some background information about
   vitamin C.
3. Ask students to bring in juices from home to
   test.

Session 3: Testing More Juices

Getting Ready
Before the Day of the Activity:
1. Remind students to bring in drinks from home.
2. Check to see that equipment and materials used in Session 1 are ready for use.
   a. Make more indophenol solution if necessary.
   b. Refill squeeze bottles.
   c. Duplicate more data sheets if necessary.
   d. (*Optional*) Duplicate graphing sheets.

The Day of the Activity:
1. Set out equipment trays for each group of 4–6 students, with cups, droppers, and tape.
2. Place all other equipment on centrally located table.
3. Arrange work stations for groups of 4–6 students.

Conducting the Tests
1. Distribute drinks students brought from home so each table has equal number.
2. Have students label and pour drinks in cups.
3. Have one member of each team get equipment and data sheets.
4. Have students test fruit drinks at their table.

Drawing Conclusions
1. Remove equipment and drinks from tables.
2. Distribute calculators and have groups average the results at each table.
3. Have representatives record results on board.
4. Discuss the results: Are there surprises? Patterns in the data? Difference between canned and fresh juices?
5. Discuss: Why might different orange juices have different vitamin C content?
6. Discuss: Are juices with equal vitamin C content equally as good?
7. (*Optional*) Copy the data off the board and distribute with graphing sheets as homework.

Session 4: Experimenting with Vitamin Content

Getting Ready
Two Days Before the Activity:
1. Buy enough oranges to make 4 cups of juice.
2. Squeeze and blend the orange juice.
3. Divide the juice in half and prepare:
   a. two cups exposed to air and left in room.
   b. two cups covered in refrigerator.
   (*Optional*) You may choose to squeeze 4 more cups and:
   c. freeze two cups.
   d. boil two cups.

The Day Before the Activity
1. Label cups.
2. Check to see that equipment and materials used in Session 1 are ready for use:
   a. Make more indophenol solution if necessary.
   b. Refill squeeze bottles.
   c. Duplicate more data sheets if necessary.
3. (*Optional*) Remove the frozen orange juice from freezer.

The Day of the Activity:
1. Replace water lost from orange juice due to evaporation.
2. Pour juices into cups, add medicine droppers, set on trays.
3. Place all other equipment on centrally located table.
4. Arrange work stations for groups of 4–6 students.
5. List the treated juices vertically on the board.

Experimenting
1. Ask why parents tell children to, "Cover the juice and put it in the refrigerator."
2. Explain how juice was treated.
3. Ask students to predict vitamin C content of each.
4. Have one member of each team get equipment and data sheets.
5. Distribute trays of juices.
6. Have students test juices.
7. Remove equipment and juices from table.

Pooling Data and Analyzing Results
1. Have students write their results on the chalkboard.
2. Assign individuals to calculate class averages.
3. Make a bar graph of the results on the chalkboard.
4. Help the students draw conclusions.
5. Provide background information about vitamin loss and retention.

Vitamin C Testing— Data Sheet

What to do:

1. Measure 10 ml indophenol and put in test vial.
2. Measure 10 ml water and put in control vial.
3. Add 1 drop of the test beverage to each vial and *stir well.*
4. Keep adding, drop by drop, until the contents in both vials look the same. Remember to stir after each drop.
5. After testing all beverages, **rank** the beverages in vitamin C content: most vitamin C = 1; second most = 2; and so on.

Indophenol Color Changes: *Blue → Violet → Pink → No Color*

Test beverages	Number of drops needed for indophenol to lose all color	Rank 1 = Most Vit. C

© 1988 by the Regents of the University of California
LHS—Great Explorations in Math and Science: *Vitamin C Testing*

Name _____

Vitamin C Testing— Graphing Sheet

Number of drops

50
49
48
47
46
45
44
43
42
41
40
39
38
37
36
35
34
33
32
31
30
29
28
27
26
25
24
23
22
21
20
19
18
17
16
15
14
13
12
11
10
9
8
7
6
5
4
3
2
1
0

Test Beverage

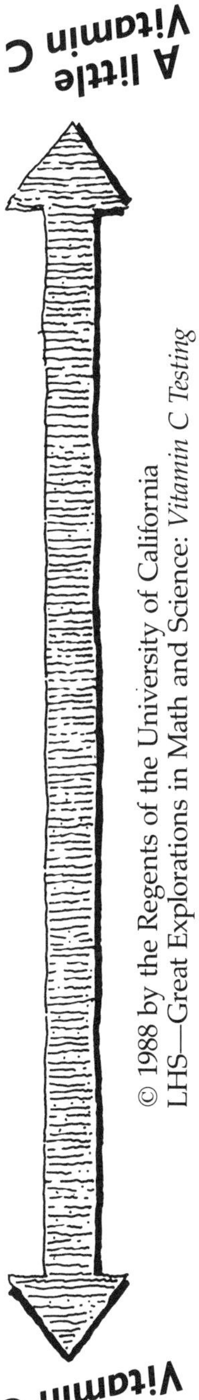

A little Vitamin C

A lot of Vitamin C

INDOPHENOL SOLUTION	INDOPHENOL SOLUTION	INDOPHENOL SOLUTION
INDOPHENOL SOLUTION	INDOPHENOL SOLUTION	INDOPHENOL SOLUTION
INDOPHENOL SOLUTION	INDOPHENOL SOLUTION	INDOPHENOL SOLUTION
INDOPHENOL SOLUTION	INDOPHENOL SOLUTION	INDOPHENOL SOLUTION
WATER	WATER	WATER
WATER	WATER	WATER
WATER	WATER	WATER
VITAMIN C SOLUTION	VITAMIN C SOLUTION	VITAMIN C SOLUTION
VITAMIN C SOLUTION	VITAMIN C SOLUTION	VITAMIN C SOLUTION
VITAMIN C SOLUTION	VITAMIN C SOLUTION	VITAMIN C SOLUTION

Notes

Notes